KETO CHAFFLE RECIPES

Cookbook for Beginners 2021 for a healthy life. Quick and easy waffles to cook at home with your guest and family.

TABLE OF CONTENTS

BREAKFAST CHAFFLE RECIPES

Mini Breakfast Chaffle

Preparation Time: 10 minutes
Cooking Time: 15 Minutes
Servings: 3
Ingredients:
- 6 tsp coconut flour
- 1 tsp stevia
- 1/4 tsp baking powder
- 2 eggs
- 3 oz. cream cheese
- 1/2. tsp vanilla extract

Topping
- 1 egg
- 6 slice bacon
- 2 oz. Raspberries for topping
- 2 oz. Blueberries for topping
- 2 oz. Strawberries for topping

Directions:
1. Heat up your square waffle maker and grease with cooking spray.
2. Mix together coconut flour, stevia, egg, baking powder, cheese and vanilla in mixing bowl.
3. Pour ½ of chaffles mixture in a waffle maker.

4. Close the lid and cook the chaffles for about 3-5 minutes Utes.
5. Meanwhile, fry bacon slices in pan on medium heat for about 2-3 minutes Utes until cooked and transfer them to plate.
6. In the same pan, fry eggs one by one in the leftover grease of bacon.
7. Once chaffles are cooked, carefully transfer them to plate.
8. Serve with fried eggs and bacon slice and berries on top.
9. Enjoy!

Nutrition: Calories: 480 Fat: 30 g Net Carbohydrates: 4 g Protein: 45 g

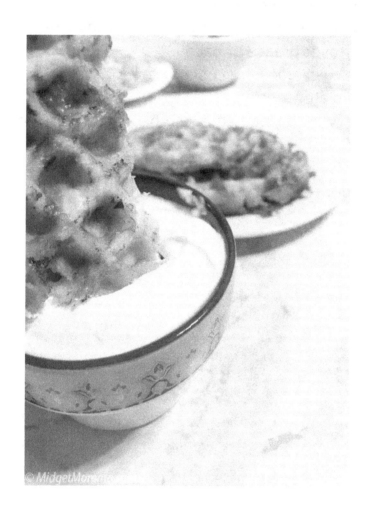

Chaffles With Egg & Asparagus

Preparation Time: 10 minutes
Cooking Time: 10 Minutes
Servings:1
Ingredients:
- 1 egg
- 1/4 cup cheddar cheese
- 2 tbsps. almond flour
- ½ tsp. baking powder

Topping
- 1 egg
- 4-5 stalks asparagus
- 1 tsp avocado oil

Directions:
1. Preheat waffle maker to medium-high heat.
2. Whisk together egg, mozzarella cheese, almond flour, and baking powder
3. Pour chaffles mixture into the center of the waffle iron. Close the waffle maker and let cook for 5 minutes Utes or until waffle is golden brown and set.
4. Remove chaffles from the waffle maker and serve.
5. Meanwhile, heat oil in a nonstick pan.
6. Once the pan is hot, fry asparagus for about 4-5 minutes Utes until golden brown.
7. Poach the egg in boil water for about 2-3 minutes Utes.

8. Once chaffles are cooked, remove from the maker.
9. Serve chaffles with the poached egg and asparagus.

Nutrition: Calories: 843 Total Fat: 65g Saturated Fat: 14g Protein: 59g

Cholesterol: 156mg Carbohydrates: 6g Fiber: 1g Net Carbs: 5g

Delicious Raspberries taco Chaffles

Preparation Time: 10 minutes
Cooking Time: 15 Minutes
Servings:1
Ingredients:
- 1 egg white
- 1/4 cup jack cheese, shredded
- 1/4 cup cheddar cheese, shredded
- 1 tsp coconut flour
- 1/4 tsp baking powder
- 1/2 tsp stevia

For Topping
- 4 oz. raspberries
- 2 tbsps. coconut flour
- 2 oz. unsweetened raspberry sauce

Directions:
1. Switch on your round Waffle Maker and grease it with cooking spray once it is hot.
2. Mix together all chaffle ingredients in a bowl and combine with a fork.
3. Pour chaffle batter in a preheated maker and close the lid.
4. Roll the taco chaffle around using a kitchen roller, set it aside and allow it to set for a few minutes Utes.
5. Once the taco chaffle is set, remove from the roller.
6. Dip raspberries in sauce and arrange on taco chaffle.

7. Drizzle coconut flour on top.

8. Enjoy raspberries taco chaffle with keto coffee.

Nutrition: Protein: 28% 77 kcal Fat: 6 187 kcal Carbohydrates: 3% 8 kcal

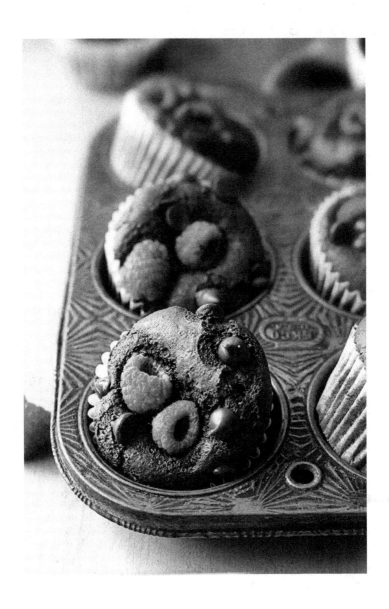

Coconut Chaffles with Boiled Egg

Preparation Time: 10 minutes
Cooking Time: 5 Minutes
Servings:2
Ingredients:
- 1 egg
- 1 oz. cream cheese,
- 1 oz. cheddar cheese
- 2 tbsps. coconut flour
- 1 tsp. stevia
- 1 tbsp. coconut oil, melted
- 1/2 tsp. coconut extract
- 2 eggs, soft boil for serving

Directions:
1. Heat you minutes Dash waffle maker and grease with cooking spray.
2. Mix together all chaffles ingredients in a bowl.
3. Pour chaffle batter in a preheated waffle maker.
4. Close the lid.
5. Cook chaffles for about 2-3 minutes Utes until golden brown.
6. Serve with boil egg and enjoy!

Nutrition: Calories: 363 kcal Protein: 35.33 g Fat: 22.14 g Carbohydrates: 6.83 g

Garlic and Parsley Chaffle

Preparation Time: 10 minutes
Cooking Time: 5 Minutes
Servings:1
Ingredients:
- 1 large egg
- 1/4 cup cheese mozzarella
- 1 tsp. coconut flour
- ¼ tsp. baking powder
- ½ tsp. garlic powder
- 1 tbsp. minutes parsley

For Serving
- 1 Poach egg
- 4 oz. smoked salmon

Directions:
1. Switch on your Dash minutes waffle maker and let it preheat.
2. Grease waffle maker with cooking spray.
3. Mix together egg, mozzarella, coconut flour, baking powder, and garlic powder, parsley to a mixing bowl until combined well.
4. Pour batter in circle chaffle maker.
5. Close the lid.
6. Cook for about 2-3 minutes Utes or until the chaffles are cooked.
7. Serve with smoked salmon and poached egg.
8. Enjoy!

Nutrition: Protein: 45% 140 kcal Fat: 51% 160 kcal Carbohydrates: 4% 14 kcal

Scrambled Eggs on A Spring Onion Chaffle

Preparation Time: 10 minutes
Cooking Time:7–9 Minutes
Servings:4

Ingredients:
- Batter
- 4 eggs
- 2 cups grated mozzarella cheese
- 2 spring onions, finely chopped
- Salt and pepper to taste
- ½ teaspoon dried garlic powder
- 2 tablespoons almond flour
- 2 tablespoons coconut flour

Other
- 2 tablespoons butter for brushing the waffle maker
- 6-8 eggs
- Salt and pepper
- 1 teaspoon Italian spice mix
- 1 tablespoon olive oil
- 1 tablespoon freshly chopped parsley

Directions:
1. Preheat the waffle maker.
2. Crack the eggs into a bowl and add the grated cheese.
3. Mix until just combined, then add the chopped spring onions and season with salt and pepper and dried garlic powder.

---

4. Stir in the almond flour and mix until everything is combined.
5. Brush the heated waffle maker with butter and add a few tablespoons of the batter.
6. Close the lid and cook for about 7–8 minutes depending on your waffle maker.
7. While the chaffles are cooking, prepare the scrambled eggs by whisking the eggs in a bowl until frothy, about 2 minutes. Season with salt and black pepper to taste and add the Italian spice mix. Whisk to blend in the spices.
8. Warm the oil in a non-stick pan over medium heat.
9. Pour the eggs in the pan and cook until eggs are set to your liking.
10. Serve each chaffle and top with some scrambled eggs. Top with freshly chopped parsley.

Nutrition: Calories 194, fat 14.7 g, carbs 5 g, sugar 0.6 g, Protein 1 g, sodium 191 mg

Egg on A Cheddar Cheese Chaffle

Preparation Time: 10 minutes
Cooking Time:7–9 Minutes
Servings:4
Ingredients:
- Batter
- 4 eggs
- 2 cups shredded white cheddar cheese
- Salt and pepper to taste
- Other
- 2 tablespoons butter for brushing the waffle maker
- 4 large eggs
- 2 tablespoons olive oil

Directions:
1. Preheat the waffle maker.
2. Crack the eggs into a bowl and whisk them with a fork.
3. Stir in the grated cheddar cheese and season with salt and pepper.
4. Brush the heated waffle maker with butter and add a few tablespoons of the batter.
5. Close the lid and cook for about 7–8 minutes depending on your waffle maker.
6. While chaffles are cooking, cook the eggs.
7. Warm the oil in a large non-stick pan that has a lid over medium-low heat for 2-3 minutes

8. Crack an egg in a small ramekin and gently add it to the pan. Repeat the same way for the other 3 eggs.
9. Cover and let cook for 2 to 2 ½ minutes for set eggs but with runny yolks.
10. Remove from heat.
11. To serve, place a chaffle on each plate and top with an egg. Season with salt and black pepper to taste.

Nutrition: Calories 4 fat 34 g, carbs 2 g, sugar 0.6 g, Protein 26 g, sodium 518 mg

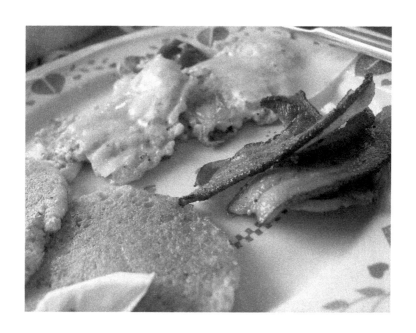

Avocado Chaffles Toast

Preparation Time: 10 minutes
Cooking Time: 10 Minutes
Servings:3
Ingredients:
- 4 tbsps. avocado mash
- 1/2 tsp lemon juice
- 1/8 tsp salt
- 1/8 tsp black pepper
- 2 eggs
- 1/2 cup shredded cheese

For serving
- 3 eggs
- ½ avocado thinly sliced
- 1 tomato, sliced

Directions:
1. Mash avocado mash with lemon juice, salt, and black pepper in mixing bowl, until well combined.
2. In a small bowl beat egg and pour eggs in avocado mixture and mix well.
3. Switch on Waffle Maker to pre-heat.
4. Pour 1/8 of shredded cheese in a waffle maker and then pour ½ of egg and avocado mixture and then 1/8 shredded cheese.
5. Close the lid and cook chaffles for about 3 - 4 minutes Utes.
6. Repeat with the remaining mixture.
7. Meanwhile, fry eggs in a pan for about 1-2 minutes Utes.

8. For serving, arrange fried egg on chaffle toast with avocado slice and tomatoes.
9. Sprinkle salt and pepper on top and enjoy!

Nutrition: Protein: 26% 66 kcal Fat: 67% 169 kcal Carbohydrates: 6% 15 kcal

Cajun & Feta Chaffle

Preparation Time: 10 minutes
Cooking Time: 10 Minutes
Servings:1
Ingredients:
- 1 egg white
- 1/4 cup shredded mozzarella cheese
- 2 tbsps. almond flour
- 1 tsp Cajun Seasoning
- FOR SERVING
- 1 egg
- 4 oz. feta cheese
- 1 tomato, sliced

Directions:
1. Whisk together egg, cheese, and seasoning in a bowl.
2. Switch on and grease waffle maker with cooking spray.
3. Pour batter in a preheated waffle maker.
4. Cook chaffles for about 2-3 minutes Utes until the chaffle is cooked through.
5. Meanwhile, fry the egg in a non-stick pan for about 1-2 minutes Utes.
6. For serving set fried egg on chaffles with feta cheese and tomatoes slice.

Nutrition: Protein: 28% 119 kcal Fat: 64% 2 kcal Carbohydrates: 7% 31 kcal

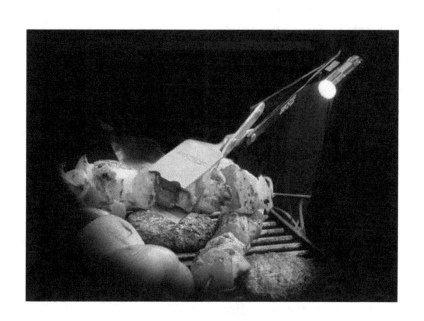

Crispy Chaffles Plus Sausage

Preparation Time: 10 minutes
Cooking Time: 10 Minutes
Servings:2
Ingredients:
- 1/2 cup cheddar cheese
- 1/2 tsp. baking powder
- 1/4 cup egg whites
- 2 tsp. pumpkin spice
- 1 egg, whole
- 2 chicken sausage
- 2 slice bacon
- salt and pepper to taste
- 1 tsp. avocado oil

Directions:
1. Mix together all ingredients in a bowl.
2. Allow batter to sit while waffle iron warms.
3. Spray waffle iron with nonstick spray.
4. Pour batter in the waffle maker and cook according to the directions of the manufacturer.
5. Meanwhile, heat oil in a pan and fry the egg, according to your choice and transfer it to plate.
6. In the same pan, fry bacon slice and sausage on medium heat for about 2-3 minutes Utes until cooked.
7. Once chaffles are cooked thoroughly, remove them from the maker.
8. Serve with fried egg, bacon slice, sausages and enjoy!

Nutrition: Protein: 22% 86 kcal Fat: 74% 286 kcal Carbohydrates: 3% 12 kcal

Chili Chaffles

Preparation Time: 10 minutes
Cooking Time: 7–9 Minutes
Servings: 4
Ingredients:
- Batter
- 4 eggs
- ½ cup grated parmesan cheese
- 1½ cups grated yellow cheddar cheese
- 1 hot red chili pepper
- Salt and pepper to taste
- ½ teaspoon dried garlic powder
- 1 teaspoon dried basil
- 2 tablespoons almond flour

Other
- 2 tablespoons olive oil for brushing the waffle maker

Directions:
1. Preheat the waffle maker.
2. Crack the eggs into a bowl and add the grated parmesan and cheddar cheese.
3. Mix until just combined and add the chopped chili pepper. Season with salt and pepper, dried garlic powder and dried basil. Stir in the almond flour.
4. Mix until everything is combined.
5. Brush the heated waffle maker with olive oil and add a few tablespoons of the batter.
6. Close the lid and cook for about 7–8 minutes depending on your waffle maker.

Nutrition: Calories 36 fat 30.4 g, carbs 3.1 g, sugar 0.7 g, Protein 21.5 g, sodium 469 mg

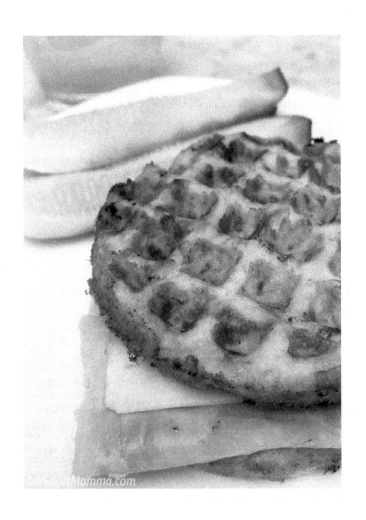

Simple & Savory Chaffle

Preparation Time: 10 minutes
Cooking Time: 7–9 Minutes
Servings:4
Ingredients:
- Batter
- 4 eggs
- 1 cup grated mozzarella cheese
- 1 cup grated provolone cheese
- ½ cup almond flour
- 2 tablespoons coconut flour
- 2½ teaspoons baking powder
- Salt and pepper to taste
- Other
- 2 tablespoons butter to brush the waffle maker

Directions:
1. Preheat the waffle maker.
2. Add the grated mozzarella and provolone cheese to a bowl and mix.
3. Add the almond and coconut flour and baking powder and season with salt and pepper.
4. Mix with a wire whisk and crack in the eggs.
5. Stir everything together until batter forms.
6. Brush the heated waffle maker with butter and add a few tablespoons of the batter.
7. Close the lid and cook for about 8 minutes depending on your waffle maker.
8. Serve and enjoy.

Nutrition: Calories 352, fat 27.2 g, carbs 8.3 g, sugar 0.5 g, Protein 15 g, sodium 442 mg

waffle

Preparation Time: 10 minutes
Cooking Time:7–9 Minutes
Servings:4

Ingredients:

- Batter
- 4 eggs
- 1½ cups grated mozzarella cheese
- ½ cup grated parmesan cheese
- 2 tablespoons tomato sauce
- ¼ cup almond flour
- 1½ teaspoons baking powder
- Salt and pepper to taste
- 1 teaspoon dried oregano
- ¼ cup sliced salami
- Other
- 2 tablespoons olive oil for brushing the waffle maker
- ¼ cup tomato sauce for serving

Directions:

1. Preheat the waffle maker.
2. Add the grated mozzarella and grated parmesan to a bowl and mix.
3. Add the almond flour and baking powder and season with salt and pepper and dried oregano.
4. Mix with a wooden spoon or wire whisk and crack in the eggs.
5. Stir everything together until batter forms.
6. Stir in the chopped salami.

7. Brush the heated waffle maker with olive oil and add a few tablespoons of the batter.
8. Close the lid and cook for about 7–minutes depending on your waffle maker.
9. Serve with extra tomato sauce on top and enjoy.

Nutrition: Calories 319, fat 25.2 g, carbs 5.9 g, sugar 1.7 g, Protein 19.3 g, sodium 596 mg

Breakfast Bacon Chaffles

Preparation Time: 10 minutes
Cooking Time:7–9 Minutes
Servings:4
Ingredients:
- Batter
- 4 eggs
- 2 cups shredded mozzarella
- 2 ounces finely chopped bacon
- Salt and pepper to taste
- 1 teaspoon dried oregano
- Other
- 2 tablespoons olive oil for brushing the waffle maker

Directions:
1. Preheat the waffle maker.
2. Crack the eggs into a bowl and add the grated mozzarella cheese.
3. Mix until just combined and stir in the chopped bacon.
4. Season with salt and pepper and dried oregano.
5. Brush the heated waffle maker with olive oil and add a few tablespoons of the batter.
6. Close the lid and cook for about 7–8 minutes depending on your waffle maker.

Nutrition: Calories 241, fat 19.8 g, carbs 1.3 g, sugar 0.4 g, Protein 14.8 g, sodium 4 mg

Chaffles Bowl

Preparation Time: 10 minutes
Cooking Time: 5 Minutes
Servings:2

Ingredients:
- 1 egg
- 1/2 cup cheddar cheese shredded
- pinch of Italian seasoning
- 1 tbsp. pizza sauce
- TOPPING
- 1/2 avocado sliced
- 2 eggs boiled
- 1 tomato, halves
- 4 oz. fresh spinach leaves

Directions:
1. Preheat your waffle maker and grease with cooking spray.
2. Crack an egg in a small bowl and beat with Italian seasoning and pizza sauce.
3. Add shredded cheese to the egg and spices mixture.
4. Pour 1 tbsp. shredded cheese in a waffle maker and cook for 30 sec.
5. Pour Chaffles batter in the waffle maker and close the lid.
6. Cook chaffles for about 4 minutes Utes until crispy and brown.
7. Carefully remove chaffles from the maker.

8. Serve on the bed of spinach with boil egg, avocado slice, and tomatoes.
9. Enjoy!

Nutrition: Protein: 23% 77 kcal Fat: 66% 222 kcal Carbohydrates: 11% 39 kcal

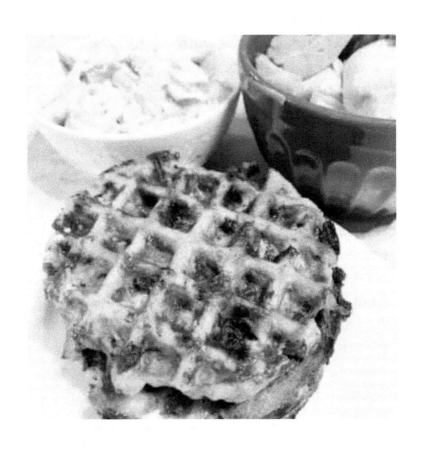

Morning Chaffles With Berries

Preparation Time: 10 minutes
Cooking Time: 5 Minutes
Servings: 4
Ingredients:
- 1 cup egg whites
- 1 cup cheddar cheese, shredded
- ¼ cup almond flour
- ¼ cup heavy cream
- TOPPING
- 4 oz. raspberries
- 4 oz. strawberries.
- 1 oz. keto chocolate flakes
- 1 oz. feta cheese.

Directions:
1. Preheat your square waffle maker and grease with cooking spray.
2. Beat egg white in a small bowl with flour.
3. Add shredded cheese to the egg whites and flour mixture and mix well.
4. Add cream and cheese to the egg mixture.
5. Pour Chaffles batter in a waffle maker and close the lid.
6. Cook chaffles for about 4 minutes Utes until crispy and brown.
7. Carefully remove chaffles from the maker.
8. Serve with berries, cheese, and chocolate on top.
9. Enjoy!

Nutrition: Protein: 28% 68 kcal Fat: 67% 163 kcal
Carbohydrates: 5% 12 kcal

Mixed Berry & Vanilla Chaffles

Preparation time: 10 minutes
Cooking time: 28 minutes
Servings: 4
Ingredients:
- 1 egg, beaten
- ½ cup finely grated mozzarella cheese
- 1 tbsp cream cheese, softened
- 1 tbsp sugar-free maple syrup
- 2 strawberries, sliced
- 2 raspberries, slices
- ¼ tsp blackberry extract
- ¼ tsp vanilla extract
- ½ cup plain yogurt for serving

Directions:
1. Preheat the waffle iron.
2. In a medium bowl, mix all the ingredients except the yogurt.
3. Open the iron, lightly grease with cooking spray and pour in a quarter of the mixture.
4. Close the iron and cook until golden brown and crispy, 7 minutes.
5. Remove the chaffle onto a plate and set aside.
6. Make three more chaffles with the remaining mixture.
7. To serve: top with the yogurt and enjoy.

Nutrition: Calories: 99 Cal Total Fat: 8 g Saturated Fat: 0 g Cholesterol: 0 mg Sodium: 0 mg Total Carbs: 4 g

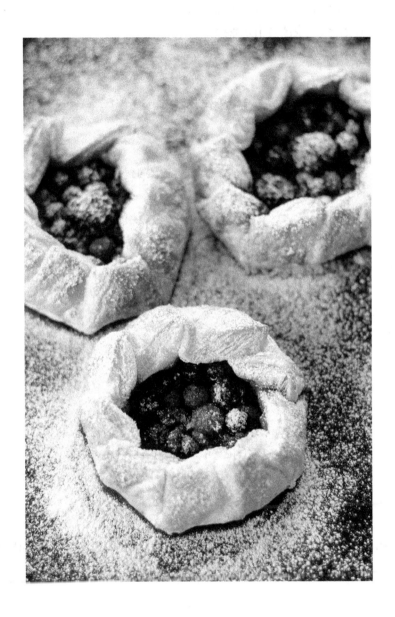

Ham and Cheddar Chaffles

Preparation time: 15 minutes
Cooking time: 28 minutes
Servings: 4
Ingredients:
- 1 cup finely shredded parsnips, steamed
- 8 oz ham, diced
- 2 eggs, beaten
- 1 ½ cups finely grated cheddar cheese
- ½ tsp garlic powder
- 2 tbsp chopped fresh parsley leaves
- ¼ tsp smoked paprika
- ½ tsp dried thyme
- Salt and freshly ground black pepper to taste

Directions:
1. Preheat the waffle iron.
2. In a medium bowl, mix all the ingredients.
3. Open the iron, lightly grease with cooking spray and pour in a quarter of the mixture.
4. Close the iron and cook until crispy, 7 minutes.
5. Remove the chaffle onto a plate and set aside.
6. Make three more chaffles using the remaining mixture.
7. Serve afterward.

Nutrition: Calories: 99 Cal Total Fat: 8 g Saturated Fat: 0 g Cholesterol: 0 mg Sodium: 0 mg Total Carbs: 4 g

Savory Gruyere and Chives Chaffles

Preparation time: 15 minutes
Cooking time: 14 minutes
Servings: 2
Ingredients:

- 2 eggs, beaten
- 1 cup finely grated Gruyere cheese
- 2 tbsp finely grated cheddar cheese
- 1/8 tsp freshly ground black pepper
- 3 tbsp minced fresh chives + more for garnishing
- 2 sunshine fried eggs for topping

Directions:

1. Preheat the waffle iron.
2. In a medium bowl, mix the eggs, cheeses, black pepper, and chives.
3. Open the iron and pour in half of the mixture.
4. Close the iron and cook until brown and crispy, 7 minutes.
5. Remove the chaffle onto a plate and set aside.
6. Make another chaffle using the remaining mixture.
7. Top each chaffle with one fried egg each, garnish with the chives and serve.

Nutrition: Calories: 99 Cal Total Fat: 8 g Saturated Fat: 0 g Cholesterol: 0 mg Sodium: 0 mg Total Carbs: 4 g

Chicken Quesadilla Chaffle

Preparation time: 10 minutes
Cooking time: 14 minutes
Servings: 2

Ingredients:
- 1 egg, beaten
- ¼ tsp taco seasoning
- 1/3 cup finely grated cheddar cheese
- 1/3 cup cooked chopped chicken

Directions:
1. Preheat the waffle iron.
2. In a medium bowl, mix the eggs, taco seasoning, and cheddar cheese. Add the chicken and combine well.
3. Open the iron, lightly grease with cooking spray and pour in half of the mixture.
4. Close the iron and cook until brown and crispy, 7 minutes.
5. Remove the chaffle onto a plate and set aside.
6. Make another chaffle using the remaining mixture.
7. Serve afterward.

Nutrition: Calories: 99 Cal Total Fat: 8 g Saturated Fat: 0 g Cholesterol: 0 mg Sodium: 0 mg Total Carbs: 4 g

BASIC CHAFFLE RECIPES

Chaffle Chicken Breast Stuffed with Spinach, Pine Nuts, and Feta

Preparation time:20 minutes
Cooking time: 15 minutes
Serving: 4-6
Ingredients
- 1 cup finely chopped fresh baby spinach
- 3/4 cup feta cheese, crumbled
- 2 tablespoons toasted pine nuts
- 2 cloves garlic, minced
- ½ teaspoon dried thyme
- 4 boneless, skinless chicken breast halves
- ½ teaspoon salt
- ½ teaspoon freshly ground black pepper

NOTE: The Use of baby spinach reduces the stress of picking through to remove large stems.
The use of toasted pine nut is to bring out the flavor.

Directions:
1. Toasting the pine nut
2. Put the pine nuts inside a dry pan over medium heat.
3. Stir frequently till the nuts become fragrant and are barely turning brown.
4. Remove from the heat and pour them onto a plate to cool.

Making the Chaffles

1. Preheat the waffle iron and oven on medium.
2. Put the spinach, cheese, nuts, garlic, and thyme in a small bowl.
3. Smash together until the filling becomes cohesive and easier to handle.
4. Lightly grease the waffle iron
5. Make a parallel cut into the thickest portion of each chicken breast half to form a pocket. But do not to cut through.
6. Divide the combination into four equal parts and fill up each pocket in the chicken breasts, leaving a margin at the edge to close.
7. Season the chicken with salt and pepper.
8. Arrange the chicken into the waffle iron to allow lid to press down on the chicken more evenly.
9. Close the lid.
10. Cooking the chicken for 8 minutes. Check and rotate if need be and cooking for about 3 minutes. The chicken should be golden brown.
11. Remove the chicken from the waffle iron
12. Repeat baking procedure with any remaining chicken.
13. Keep cooked chicken warm and serve warm.

Nutrition: Calories 158, Fat 13.3, Fiber 3.9, Carbs 8.9, Protein 3.3

Light & Crispy Bacon Cheddar Chaffles Recipe

Preparation time: 5 minutes
Cooking time: 5 minutes
Servings: 4
Ingredients
- 2 eggs
- 1 cup cheddar
- ½ Coconut/almond flour
- 1/2 teaspoon baking powder
- Bacon
- Shredded parmesan cheese on top and bottom.

Directions:
1. Heat up the waffle iron on medium.
2. Mix eggs, cheddar cheese in a small bowl.
3. Whisk egg thoroughly
4. Mix flour, baking powder, salt together in a large bowl
5. Gently whisk the egg mixture into the dry ingredients.
6. Whisk thoroughly until smooth
7. Add the bacon into the mixture and mix thoroughly
8. Lightly grease the waffle iron
9. Ladle the batter into the waffle maker
10. Bake till crispy and golden brown.
11. Repeat baking procedure till batter is finished.
12. Serve warm.

Nutrition: Calories 129, Fat 11.7, Fiber 2.7, Carbs 5.8, Protein 2.2

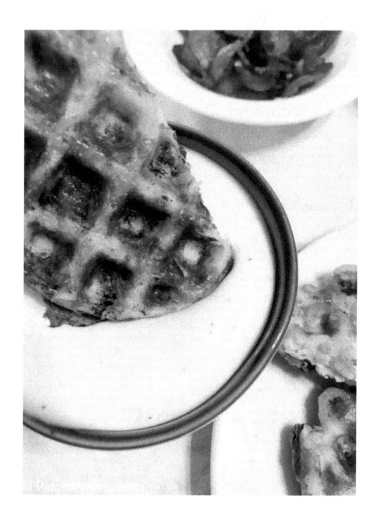

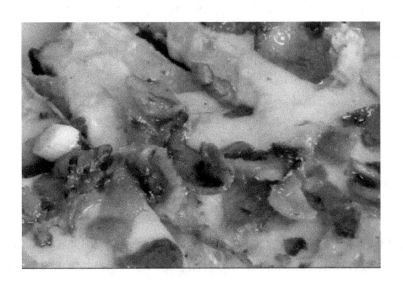

Stuffed Chaffles

Preparation time: 15 minutes
Cooking time: 15 minutes
Servings: 6
Ingredients:
- 1 tablespoon extra-virgin olive oil
- 1/4 cup chopped onion
- ½ cup chopped celery
- ¾ teaspoon salt ½ teaspoon freshly ground black pepper
- ½ teaspoon poultry seasoning
- ¼ teaspoon dried sage
- 6 cups low-carb dry bread cubes (about ½-inch square)
- ½ cup unsalted butter, melted
- 1 cup low-sodium chicken broth
- 1 cup cheese
- 4 eggs (separated)

NOTE: Cut any slightly stale pieces or ends into cubes and leave at room temperature for an hour before using.

Directions:
1. Put the bread cubes in a bowl preferably big size.
2. Mix butter, cheese, egg white and chicken broth together in a medium bowl
3. In another bowl, mix all vegetables together
4. Pour the butter mixture over the bread.
5. Add the vegetable mixture and stir.

6. Leave the stuffing mixture to sit for 5 minutes to completely absorb the liquid, stir it once or twice.
7. Preheat the waffle iron on medium heat.
8. Lightly grease the waffle iron.
9. Put close to 1/2 cup of the stuffing mix on one section of the waffle iron.
10. Use enough of the mixture to slightly overstuff each section of the waffle iron.
11. Close the lid and press down to compress the stuffing.
12. Bake till golden brown and cohesive.
13. Repeat the baking procedure until all stuffing mixtures are baked.
14. Keep completed chaffles warm
15. Serve cool

Nutrition: Calories 229, Fat 19.6, Fiber 1.8, Carbs 5.9, Protein 10.9

Broccoli & Cheese Chaffles

Preparation Time: 5 minutes
Cooking Time: 8 minutes
Servings: 2

Ingredients:
- ¼ cup broccoli florets
- 1 egg, beaten
- 1 tablespoon almond flour
- ¼ teaspoon garlic powder
- ½ cup cheddar cheese

Directions:
1. Preheat your waffle maker.
2. Add the broccoli to the food processor.
3. Pulse until chopped.
4. Add to a bowl.
5. Stir in the egg and the rest of the ingredients.
6. Mix well.
7. Pour half of the batter to the waffle maker.
8. Cover and cooking for 4 minutes.
9. Repeat procedure to make the next chaffle.

Nutrition: Calories 107, Fat 5.4, Fiber 5.6, Carbs 10, Protein 6.8

Chaffle with Sausage Gravy

Preparation Time: 5 minutes
Cooking Time: 15 minutes
Servings: 2
Ingredients:
- ¼ cup sausage, cooked
- 3 tablespoons chicken broth
- 2 teaspoons cream cheese
- 2 tablespoons heavy whipping cream
- ¼ teaspoon garlic powder
- Pepper to taste
- 2 basic chaffles

Directions:
1. Add the sausage, broth, cream cheese, cream, garlic powder and pepper to a pan over medium heat.
2. Bring to a boil and then reduce heat.
3. Simmer for 10 minutes or until the sauce has thickened.
4. Pour the gravy on top of the basic chaffles
5. Serve.

Nutrition: Calories 190, Fat 17, Fiber 5.6, Carbs 10, Protein 2.5

Crispy Keto Chaffle Bags

Preparation time: 30 minutes
Cooking time: 10 minutes
Servings: 14

Ingredients

- 90g stevia erythritol (sweetness 1: 1 like sugar)
- pieces of sweetener tabs (sweetness per tab 6g sugar)
- 100g almond flour
- 250ml unsweetened almond milk (I use alpro)
- 15g locust bean gum
- drops of vanilla flavor
- Melt 70g butter
- 5g coconut flour
- 40g protein powder vanilla (I use sportness from DM)
- 15g egg white powder

Directions:

1. Finely grind the stevia erythritol and sweetener tabs. Stir the sweet mix into the melted butter.
2. Stir in the almond milk with a whisk. Now mix in almond flour, coconut flour, egg white and egg white powder and vanilla flavor.
3. Finally, sift carob flour over it and quickly work into the mixture.
4. Let the chaffle batter rest for about 10 minutes. In the meantime, preheat the croissant machine at the highest level.

5. Now reduce the temperature a little and place 1 to 1.5 tablespoons of the chaffle batter in the middle of the hot plate and spread lightly. Carefully close the lid and wait briefly (approx. 20 seconds) until the mass "bakes on" something.
6. Now push the lid all the way down, so that the dough spreads even further. After about 1 to 1 1/2 minutes, carefully remove the chaffle with a spatula from the croissant machine and place it on a worktop lined with baking paper.
7. Wait a moment - be careful, the chaffle is hot! After half a minute at the latest, place the chaffle over the chaffle cone and roll the cone gently back and forth and press the chaffle onto the overlapping ends. Let the chaffle cool down on the cone (it only takes so long until the next chaffle is baked, i.e., at the most 2 minutes.)
8. Bake more chaffles with the rest of the dough and either form a croissant (with a cone) or chaffle cups by pouring the hot chaffle over an upturned coffee cup and pressing it down all around.
9. Let chaffles cool and serve either with ice cream or any other filling as desired.
10. If you like, you can refine the wafers with chocolate - either dip the top / bottom ends in chocolate and sprinkle with coconut flakes or grated nuts, or brush the chaffle cups with melted chocolate.
11. This brings an additional taste kick and prevents soaking

Nutrition: Calories 195, Fat 12.2, Fiber 4.2, Carbs 13.1, Protein 6.7

Pumpkin Keto Protein Pumpkin Vanilla

Preparation time: 30 minutes
Cooking time: 10 minutes
Servings: 6

Ingredients

- 1 egg
- 1 tablespoon of vanilla erythrite, passed through a sieve
- 1 pinch of cinnamon
- 15 grams of almond flour, passed through a sieve
- 1 teaspoon of baking soda
- 120 grams of mozzarella, grated
- 50 grams of Hokkaido pumpkin, grated

Directions:

1. the chaffle maker and switch it on so that it can preheat
2. In a small bowl, whisk the egg with the vanilla and cinnamon.
3. Gradually add baking soda and almond flour. I always sift it into the mix because I only work with the whisk. The recipe is so easy and there is no need to get any equipment dirty.
4. Now add the Mozzarella to the egg-flour mixture and stir with a fork until the cheese is well covered.
5. Finally, stir in the pumpkin.
6. Bake the chaffles in 2 portions over medium heat. The recipe makes 2 chaffles for my heart chaffle

maker. The dough does not stick anywhere in me even without fat, even with lean mozzarella.

7. You should consume the finished chaffles immediately. For this reason, I personally make only half the recipe when my husband is not at home. You can't taste the cheese directly hot from the iron - I don't think my husband even suspects that I could make an omelet filled with grated pumpkin and cheese.

8. When warming up in the microwave or in the two asters, a slight taste of cheese reappears.

9. So maybe cut the recipe in half! Fresh tastes best.

Nutrition: Calories 336, Fat 13.7, Fiber 2.6, Carbs 3.5, Protein 16.5

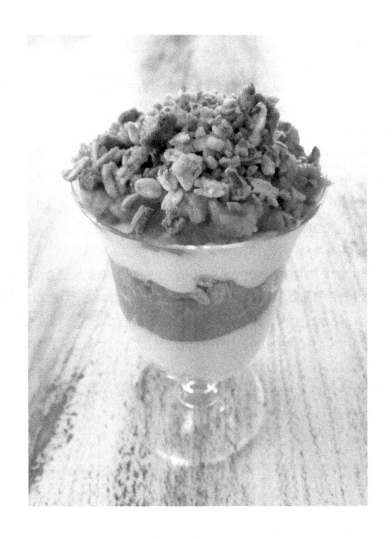

Basic Recipe for Cheese Chaffles

Preparation time: 40 minutes
Cooking time: 15 minutes
Servings: 2
Ingredients
- 1 medium or large egg
- 50 g of grated Mozzarella (fresh, self-grated is less suitable) cheese butter
- Salt
- Pepper

Directions:
1. While the chaffle iron is heating, whisk the egg and then fold in the fresh mozzarella.
2. Season with pepper and salt and add a little butter to the iron. As soon as it is melted and well distributed, add the dough and bake the cheese chaffles until they are golden brown and crispy. Salty chaffles of this type taste both warm and cold.

Nutrition: Calories 126, Fat 4.3, Fiber 2.1, Carbs 9.1, Protein 5.2

Hearty Chaffle Dough with Jalapeno

Preparation time: 10 minutes
Cooking time: 5 minutes
Servings: 2

Ingredients
- 3 large eggs
- 2 to 3 jalapenos, cored, one diced, the other cut into strips
- 4 slices of bacon
- 225 g cream cheese
- 115 g grated cheddar cheese
- 3 tbsp. coconut flour
- 1 teaspoon Baking powder
- 1/4 tsp. Himalayan salt

Directions:
1. Fry the bacon until crispy in a pan. In the meantime, mix the dry ingredients together and beat the cream cheese in a separate bowl until creamy. Heat the chaffle iron and grease it. Whisk the eggs and fold in half of the cream cheese and cheese, then the dry ingredients. Finally, fold in the diced jalapenos.
2. Bake the cheese wafers by putting half of the dough in the iron, taking out the chaffle after about 5 minutes and then baking the other half.
3. Serve the chaffles with the rest of the cream cheese, the bacon and the remaining jalapenos.

Nutrition: Calories 137, Fat 7.9, Fiber 2.3, Carbs 5.1, Protein 7.2

Cheese Chaffle Recipe with Cinnamon, Vanilla & Almond Flour

Preparation time: 10 minutes
Cooking time: 5 minutes
Servings: 2

Ingredients

- 1 egg
- 115 g grated Mozzarella
- 1 tbsp. almond flour
- 1 teaspoon Baking powder
- 1 tsp. vanilla extract
- 1 pinch of cinnamon Fat for the chaffle maker

Directions:

1. Mix the egg with the vanilla extract.
2. Mix the dry ingredients in a separate bowl and add them to the egg.
3. Finally, fold in the cheese, grease the chaffle iron and pour half of the dough into it.
4. Now bake the chaffle for about 5 minutes or until it is golden brown and crispy.
5. Check periodically so that it doesn't burn.
6. Repeat with the other half of the batter and serve the still warm chaffles with a little butter and low-carb syrup as you like.

Nutrition: Calories 278, Fat 8.3, Fiber 4.3, Carbs 8.8, Protein 23.7

Keto Chocolate Twinkie Copycat Chaffle

Preparation time: 5 minutes
Cooking time: 12 minutes
Servings: 3
Ingredients

- 2 tablespoons of butter (cooled)
- 2 oz. cream cheese softened
- Two large egg room temperature
- 1 teaspoon of vanilla essence
- 1/4 cup Lacanto confectionery
- Pinch of pink salt
- 1/4 cup almond flour
- 2 tablespoons coconut powder
- 2 tablespoons cocoa powder
- 1 teaspoon baking powder

Directions:

1. Preheat the Maker of Corndog.
2. Melt the butter for a minute and let it cool.
3. In the butter, whisk the eggs until smooth.
4. Remove sugar, cinnamon, sweetener and blend well.
5. Add flour of almond, flour of coconut, powder of cacao and baking powder.
6. Blend until well embedded.
7. Fill each well with ~2 tablespoons of batter and spread evenly.
8. Close the lid and let it cooking for 4 minutes.
9. Lift from the rack and cool it down.

Nutrition: Calories 202, Fat 6.6, Fiber 5,.4, Carbs 2.9, Protein 9.2

Easy Corndog Chaffle Recipe

Preparation time: 10 minutes
Cooking time: 4 minutes
Servings: 5
Ingredients:
- 2 eggs
- 1 cup Mexican cheese blend
- 1 tbs almond flour
- 1/2 tsp. cornbread extract
- 1/4 tsp. salt
- hot dogs with hot dog sticks

Directions:
1. Preheat corndog waffle maker.
2. In a small bowl, whip the eggs.
3. Add the remaining ingredients except the hotdogs
4. Spray the corndog waffle maker with non-stick cooking spray.
5. Fill the corndog waffle maker with the batter halfway filled.
6. Place a stick in the hot dog.
7. Place the hot dog in the batter and slightly press down.
8. Spread a small amount of better on top of the hot dog, just enough to fill it.
9. Makes about 4 to 5 chaffle corndogs
10. Cooking the corndog chaffles for about 4 minutes or until golden brown.
11. When done, they will easily remove from the corndog waffle maker with a pair of tongs.

12. Serve with mustard, mayo, or sugar-free ketchup!

Nutrition: Calories 304, Fat 8.3, Fiber 4.5, Carbs 1.6, Protein 7

Krispy Kreme Copycat of Glazed Raspberry Jelly-Filled Donut

Preparation time: 10 minutes
Cooking time: 3 minutes
Servings: 4

Ingredients:
- 1 egg
- 1/4 cup Mozzarella cheese shredded
- 2 T cream cheese softened
- 1 T sweetener
- 1 T almond flour
- 1/2 tsp. Baking Powder
- 20 drops glazed donut flavoring

Raspberry Jelly Filling Ingredients:
- 1/4 cup raspberries
- 1 tsp. chia seeds
- 1 tsp. confectioners' sweetener

Donut Glaze Ingredients
- 1 tsp. powdered sweetener
- A few drops of water or heavy whipping cream

Directions:
1. Mix everything together to make the chaffles first.
2. Cooking for about 2 1/2-3 minutes.
3. Make the Raspberry Jelly Filling:
4. Mix together in a small pot on medium heat.
5. Gently mash raspberries.
6. Let cool.
7. Add between the layers of Chaffles.

Make the Donut Glaze:
1. Stir together in a small dish.
2. Drizzle on top Chaffle.

Nutrition: Calories 186, Fat 12.1, Fiber 4.6, Carbs 11.2, Protein 7.5

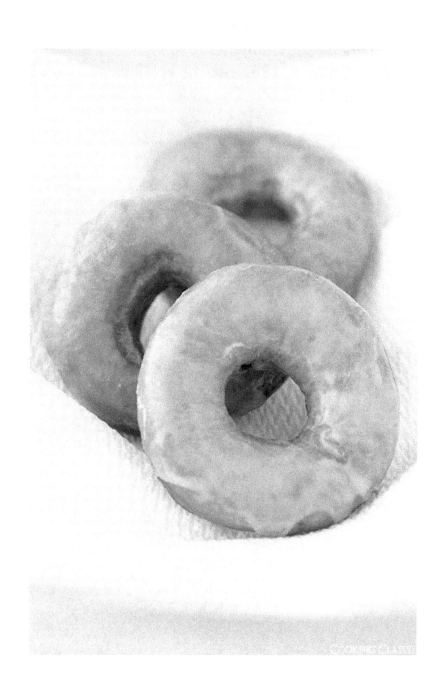

Rice Krispy Treat Chaffle Copycat Recipe

Preparation time: 15 minutes
Cooking time: 5 minutes
Servings: 2
Ingredients:
Chaffle batter:
- 1 Large Egg room temp
- 2 oz. Cream Cheese softened
- 1/4 tsp. Pure Vanilla Extract
- 2 tbs Lakanto Confectioners Sweetener
- 1 oz. Pork Rinds crushed
- 1 tsp. Baking Powder

Marshmallow Frosting:
- 1/4 c. Heavy Whipping Cream
- 1/4 tsp. Pure Vanilla Extract
- 1 tbs Lakanto Confectioners Sweetener
- 1/2 tsp. Xanthan Gum

Directions:
1. Plug in the mini waffle maker to preheat.
2. In a medium mixing bowl- Add egg, cream cheese, and vanilla.
3. Whisk until blended well.
4. Add sweetener, crushed pork rinds, and baking powder.
5. Mix until well incorporated.
6. Sprinkle extra crushed pork rinds onto waffle maker (optional).

7. Then add about 1/4 scoop of batter over, sprinkle a bit more pork rinds.
8. Cooking 3-4 minutes, then remove and cool on a wire rack.
9. Repeat for remaining batter.

Make the Marshmallow Frosting:
1. Whip the HWC, vanilla, and confectioners until thick and fluffy.
2. Slowly sprinkle over the xanthan gum and fold until well incorporated.
3. Spread frosting over chaffles and cut as desired, then refrigerate until set.
4. Enjoy cold or warm slightly in the microwave for 10 seconds.

Nutrition: Calories 203, Fat 12.3, Fiber 3.1, Carbs 5.9, Protein 4.7

Biscuits & Gravy Chaffle Recipe

Preparation time: 10 minutes
Cooking time: 5 minutes
Servings: 4
Ingredients:
- 2 tbs Unsalted Butter melted
- 2 Large Eggs
- 1 c. Mozzarella cheese shredded
- 1 tbs Garlic minced
- drops Cornbread Extract optional
- 1/2 tbs Lakanto Confectioners optional
- 1 tbs Almond Flour
- 1/4 tsp. Granulated Onion
- 1/4 tsp. Granulated Garlic
- 1 tsp. Dried Parsley
- 1 tsp. Baking Powder
- 1 batch Keto Sausage Biscuits and Gravy Recipe

Directions:
1. Preheat Mini Waffle Maker.
2. Melt the butter, let cool.
3. Whisk in the eggs, then fold in the shredded cheese.
4. Add the rest of ingredients and mix thoroughly.
5. Scoop 1/4 of batter onto waffle maker and cooking 4 minutes.
6. Remove and let cool on wire rack.
7. Repeat for the remaining 3 chaffles.

Nutrition: Calories 270, Fat 10.1, Fiber 4.7, Carbs 6.3, Protein 5.8

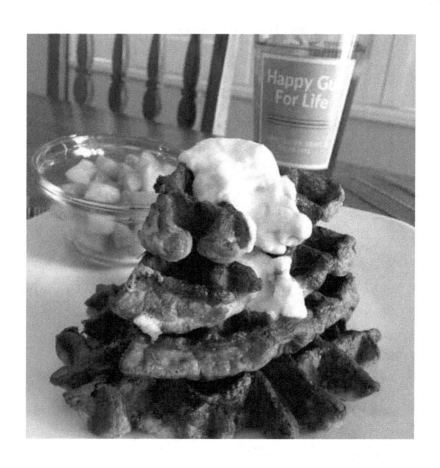

Keto Tuna Melt Chaffle Recipe

Preparation time: 15 minutes
Cooking time: 8 minutes
Servings: 2
Ingredients:
- 1 packet Tuna 2.6 oz. with no water
- 1/2 cup Mozzarella cheese
- 1 egg
- pinch salt

Directions:
1. Preheat the mini waffle maker
2. In a small bowl, add the egg and whip it up.
3. Add the tuna, cheese, and salt and mix well.
4. Optional step for an extra crispy crust: Add a teaspoon of cheese to the mini waffle maker for about 30 seconds before adding the recipe mixture. This will allow the cheese to get crispy when the tuna chaffle is done cooking. I prefer this method!
5. Add 1/2 the mixture to the waffle maker and cooking it for a minimum of 4 minutes.
6. Remove it and cooking the last tuna chaffle for another 4 minutes.

Nutrition: Calories 283, Fat 20.2, Fiber 3.3, Carbs 1.4, Protein 14.5

Blueberry & Brie Grilled Cheese Chaffle

Preparation time: 10 minutes
Cooking time: 10 minutes
Ingredients:
- 2 chaffles
- 1 t blueberry compote
- 1 oz. Wisconsin brie sliced thin
- 1 t Kerry gold butter

Chaffle Ingredients:
- 1 egg, beaten
- 1/4 cup Mozzarella shredded
- 1 tsp. Swerve confectioners
- 1 T cream cheese softened
- 1/4 tsp. baking powder
- 1/2 tsp. vanilla extract

Blueberry Compote Ingredients:
- 1 cup blueberries washed
- Zest of 1/2 lemon
- 1 T lemon juice freshly squeezed
- 1 T Swerve Confectioners
- 1/8 tsp. xanthan gum
- 2 T water

Directions:
1. Mix everything together.
2. Cooking 1/2 batter for 2 1/2- 3 minutes in the mini waffle maker
3. Repeat.
4. Let cool slightly on a cooling rack.

Blueberry Compote Directions:
1. Add everything except xanthan gum to a small saucepan. Bring to a boil, reduce heat and simmer for 5-10 minutes until it starts to thicken. Sprinkle with xanthan gum and stir well.
2. Remove from heat and let cool. Store in refrigerator until ready to use.

Grilled Cheese Directions:
1. Heat butter in a small pan over medium heat. Place Brie slices on a Chaffle and top with generous 1 T scoop of prepared blueberry compote.
2. Place sandwich in pan and grill, flipping once until waffle is golden and cheese has melted, about 2 minutes per side.

Nutrition: Calories 273, Fat 16.7, Fiber 1.5, Carbs 4.1, Protein 11.8

BBQ Chicken Chaffles

Preparation time: 3 minutes
Cooking time: 8 minutes
Servings: 2
Ingredients:
- 1/3 cup cooked chicken diced
- 1/2 cup shredded cheddar cheese
- 1 tbsp. sugar-free BBQ sauce
- 1 egg
- 1 tbsp. almond flour

Directions:
1. Heat up your Dash mini waffle maker.
2. In a small bowl, mix the egg, almond flour, BBQ sauce, diced chicken, and Cheddar Cheese.
3. Add 1/2 of the batter into your mini waffle maker and cooking for 4 minutes. If they are still a bit uncooked, leave it cooking for another 2 minutes. Then cooking the rest of the batter to make a second chaffle.
4. Do not open the waffle maker before the 4-minute mark.
5. Enjoy alone or dip in BBQ Sauce or ranch dressing!

Nutrition: Calories 301, Fat 9.7, Fiber 2.7, Carbs 5.4, Protein 15.8

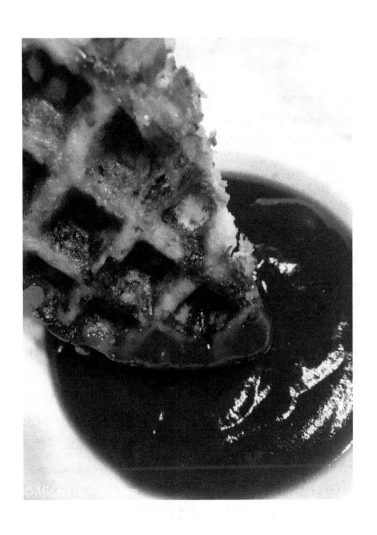

Cheddar Chicken and Broccoli Chaffle

Preparation time: 2 minutes
Cooking time: 8 minutes
Servings: 2
Ingredients:
- 1/4 cup cooked diced chicken
- 1/4 cup fresh broccoli chopped
- Shredded Cheddar cheese
- 1 egg
- 1/4 tsp. garlic powder

Directions:
1. Heat up your Dash mini waffle maker.
2. In a small bowl, mix the egg, garlic powder, and cheddar cheese.
3. Add the broccoli and chicken and mix well.
4. Add 1/2 of the batter into your mini waffle maker and cooking for 4 minutes. If they are still a bit uncooked, leave it cooking for another 2 minutes. Then cooking the rest of the batter to make a second chaffle and then cooking the third chaffle.
5. After cooking, remove from the pan and let sit for 2 minutes.
6. Dip in ranch dressing, sour cream, or enjoy alone.

Nutrition: Calories 203, Fat 12.3, Fiber 3.1, Carbs 5.9, Protein 4.7

Spinach & Artichoke Chicken Chaffle

Preparation time: 3 minutes
Cooking time: 8 minutes
Servings: 2
Ingredients:
- 1/3 cup cooked diced chicken
- 1/3 cup cooked spinach chopped
- 1/3 cup marinated artichokes chopped
- 1/3 cup shredded Mozzarella cheese
- 1-ounce softened cream cheese
- 1/4 teaspoon garlic powder
- 1 egg

Directions:
1. Heat up your Dash mini waffle maker.
2. In a small bowl, mix the egg, garlic powder, cream cheese, and Mozzarella cheese.
3. Add the spinach, artichoke, and chicken and mix well.
4. Add 1/3 of the batter into your mini waffle maker and cooking for 4 minutes. If they are still a bit uncooked, leave it cooking for another 2 minutes. Then cooking the rest of the batter to make a second chaffle and then cooking the third chaffle.
5. After cooking, remove from the pan and let sit for 2 minutes.
6. Dip in ranch dressing, sour cream, or enjoy alone.

Nutrition: Calories 126, Fat 11.2, Fiber 1.5, Carbs 2, Protein 1.5

Jamaican Jerk Chicken Chaffle

Preparation time: 5 minutes
Cooking time: 10 minutes
Servings: 4
Ingredients:
Jamaican Jerk Chicken Filling:

- 1-pound organic ground chicken browned or roasted leftover chicken finally chopped
- 2 tablespoons Kerry gold butter
- 1/2 medium onion chopped
- 1 teaspoon granulated garlic
- 1 teaspoon dried thyme
- 1/8 teaspoon black pepper
- 2 teaspoon dried parsley
- 1 teaspoon salt
- 2 teaspoon Walker's Wood Jerk Seasoning Hot and Spicy jar type paste
- 1/2 cup chicken broth

Chaffle Ingredients:

- 1/2 cup Mozzarella cheese
- 1 tablespoon butter melted
- 1 egg well beaten
- 2 tablespoon almond flour
- 1/4 teaspoon baking powder
- 1/4 teaspoon turmeric
- A pinch of xanthan gum
- A pinch of salt
- A pinch of garlic powder
- A pinch of onion powder

Directions:
1. In a medium saucepan, cooking onion in the butter.
2. Add all spices and herbs. Sauté until fragrant.
3. Add chicken.
4. Stir in chicken broth.
5. Cooking on low for 10 minutes.
6. Raise temperature to medium-high and reduce liquid until none is left in the bottom of the pan.
7. Enjoy!

Nutrition: Calories 304, Fat 24, Fiber 5.4, Carbs 6.5, Protein 13.8

CHAFFLE MEAT RECIPES

Beef Chaffle Taco

Preparation time: 10 minutes
Cooking Time:15 Minutes
Servings: 2
Ingredients:
- Batter
- 4 eggs
- 2 cups grated cheddar cheese
- ¼ cup heavy cream
- Salt and pepper to taste
- ¼ cup almond flour
- 2 teaspoons baking powder
- Beef
- 2 tablespoons butter
- ½ onion, diced
- 1 pound ground beef
- Salt and pepper to taste
- 1 teaspoon dried oregano
- 1 tablespoon sugar-free ketchup
- Other
- 2 tablespoons cooking spray to brush the waffle maker
- 2 tablespoons freshly chopped parsley

Directions:
1. Preheat the waffle maker.

2. Add the eggs, grated cheddar cheese, heavy cream, salt and pepper, almond flour and baking powder to a bowl.
3. Brush the heated waffle maker with cooking spray and add a few tablespoons of the batter.
4. Close the lid and cook for about 5–7 minutes depending on your waffle maker.
5. Once the chaffle is ready, place it in a napkin holder to harden into the shape of a taco as it cools.
6. Meanwhile, melt and heat the butter in a nonstick frying pan and start cooking the diced onion.
7. Once the onion is tender, add the ground beef. Season with salt and pepper and dried oregano and stir in the sugar-free ketchup.
8. Cook for about 7 minutes.
9. Serve the cooked ground meat in each taco chaffle sprinkled with some freshly chopped parsley.

Nutrition: Calories: 324, Fat: 20 g, Protein: 9 g, Carbohydrates: 27 g, Fiber: 1.8 g

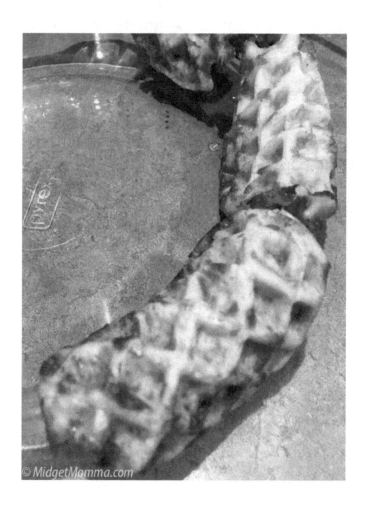

Ground Chicken Chaffle

Preparation time: 10 minutes
Cooking Time:8–10 Minutes
Servings: 2
Ingredients:
- Batter
- ½ pound ground chicken
- 4 eggs
- 3 tablespoons tomato sauce
- Salt and pepper to taste
- 1 cup grated mozzarella cheese
- 1 teaspoon dried oregano
- Other
- 2 tablespoons butter to brush the waffle maker

Directions:
1. Preheat the waffle maker.
2. Add the ground chicken, eggs and tomato sauce to a bowl and season with salt and pepper.
3. Mix everything with a fork and stir in the mozzarella cheese and dried oregano.
4. Mix again until fully combined.
5. Brush the heated waffle maker with butter and add a few tablespoons of the batter.
6. Close the lid and cook for about 8–10 minutes depending on your waffle maker.
7. Serve and enjoy.

Nutrition: Calories: 282, Fat: 16 g, Protein: 13 g, Carbohydrates: 22 g, Fiber: 3.5 g

Turkey Chaffle Sandwich

Preparation time: 10 minutes
Cooking Time:15 Minutes
Servings: 2

Ingredients:
- Batter
- 4 eggs
- ¼ cup cream cheese
- 1 cup grated mozzarella cheese
- Salt and pepper to taste
- 1 teaspoon dried dill
- ½ teaspoon onion powder
- ½ teaspoon garlic powder
- Juicy chicken
- 2 tablespoons butter
- 1 pound chicken breast
- Salt and pepper to taste
- 1 teaspoon dried dill
- 2 tablespoons heavy cream
- Other
- 2 tablespoons butter to brush the waffle maker
- 4 lettuce leaves to garnish the sandwich
- 4 tomato slices to garnish the sandwich

Directions:
1. Preheat the waffle maker.
2. Add the eggs, cream cheese, mozzarella cheese, salt and pepper, dried dill, onion powder and garlic powder to a bowl.
3. Mix everything with a fork just until batter forms.

4. Brush the heated waffle maker with butter and add a few tablespoons of the batter.
5. Close the lid and cook for about 7 minutes depending on your waffle maker.
6. Meanwhile, heat some butter in a nonstick pan.
7. Season the chicken with salt and pepper and sprinkle with dried dill. Pour the heavy cream on top.
8. Cook the chicken slices for about 10 minutes or until golden brown.
9. Cut each chaffle in half.
10.   On one half add a lettuce leaf, tomato slice, and chicken slice. Cover with the other chaffle half to make a sandwich.
11.   Serve and enjoy.

Nutrition: Calories: 102, Fat: 3 g, Protein: 9 g, Carbohydrates: 9 g, Fiber: 3.8 g

BBQ Sauce Pork Chaffle

Preparation time: 10 minutes
Cooking Time:15 Minutes
Servings: 2
Ingredients:
- ½ pound ground pork
- 3 eggs
- 1 cup grated mozzarella cheese
- Salt and pepper to taste
- 1 clove garlic, minced
- 1 teaspoon dried rosemary
- 3 tablespoons sugar-free BBQ sauce
- Other
- 2 tablespoons butter to brush the waffle maker
- ½ pound pork rinds for serving
- ¼ cup sugar-free BBQ sauce for serving

Directions:
1. Preheat the waffle maker.
2. Add the ground pork, eggs, mozzarella, salt and pepper, minced garlic, dried rosemary, and BBQ sauce to a bowl.
3. Mix until combined.
4. Brush the heated waffle maker with butter and add a few tablespoons of the batter.
5. Close the lid and cook for about 7–8 minutes depending on your waffle maker.
6. Serve each chaffle with some pork rinds and a tablespoon of BBQ sauce.

Nutrition: Calories: 225, Fat: 13 g, Protein: 12 g, Carbohydrates:15 g, Fiber: 4.3 g

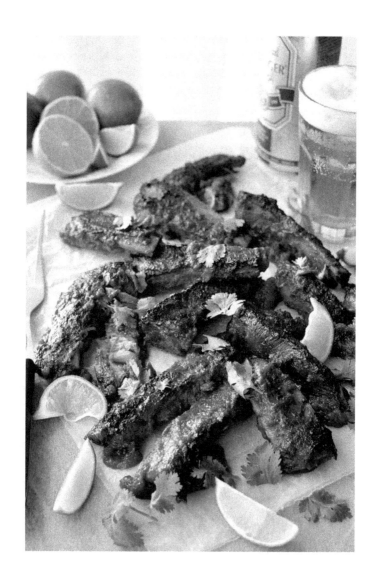

Garlic Chicken Chaffle

Preparation time: 10 minutes
Cooking Time:15 Minutes
Servings: 2
Ingredients:
- Batter
- 4 eggs
- 2 cups grated mozzarella cheese
- ¼ cup almond flour
- 2 tablespoons coconut flour
- 2½ teaspoons baking powder
- Salt and pepper to taste
- Garlic Chicken Topping
- 1-pound diced chicken
- Salt and pepper to taste
- 1 teaspoon dried oregano
- 2 garlic cloves, minced
- 3 tablespoons butter
- Other
- 2 tablespoons cooking spray for greasing the waffle maker
- 2 tablespoons freshly chopped parsley

Directions:
1. Preheat the waffle maker.
2. Add the eggs, grated mozzarella cheese, almond flour, coconut flour and baking powder to a bowl and season with salt and pepper.
3. Mix until just combined.

4. Spray the waffle maker with cooking spray to prevent the chaffles from sticking. Add a few tablespoons of the batter to the heated and greased waffle maker.
5. Close the lid and cook for about 7 minutes depending on your waffle maker.
6. Repeat with the rest of the batter.
7. Meanwhile, melt the butter in a nonstick pan over medium heat.
8. Season the chicken with salt and pepper and dried oregano and mix in the minced garlic.
9. Cook the chicken for about 10 minutes, stirring constantly.
10. Serve each chaffle with a topping of the garlic chicken mixture and sprinkle some freshly chopped parsley on top.

Nutrition: Calories: 80, Fat: 5 g, Protein: 7 g, Carbohydrates: 1 g, Fiber – 0.1 g

Chicken Taco Chaffle

Preparation time: 10 minutes
Cooking Time:15 Minutes
Servings: 2
Ingredients:
- Batter
- 4 eggs
- 2 cups grated provolone cheese
- 6 tablespoons almond flour
- 2½ teaspoons baking powder
- Salt and pepper to taste
- Chicken topping
- 2 tablespoons olive oil
- ½ pound ground chicken
- Salt and pepper to taste
- 1 garlic clove, minced
- 2 teaspoons dried oregano
- Other
- 2 tablespoons butter to brush the waffle maker
- 2 tablespoons freshly chopped spring onion for garnishing

Directions:
1. Preheat the waffle maker.
2. Add the eggs, grated provolone cheese, almond flour, baking powder and salt and pepper to a bowl.
3. Mix until just combined.
4. Brush the heated waffle maker with cooking spray and add a few tablespoons of the batter.

5. Close the lid and cook for about 7–9 minutes depending on your waffle maker.
6. Meanwhile, heat the olive oil in a nonstick pan over medium heat and start cooking the ground chicken.
7. Season with salt and pepper and stir in the minced garlic and dried oregano. Cook for 10 minutes.
8. Add some of the cooked ground chicken to each chaffle and serve with freshly chopped spring onion.

Nutrition: Calories: 366, Fat: 18 g, Protein: 18 g, Carbohydrates: 33 g, Fiber: 2.5 g

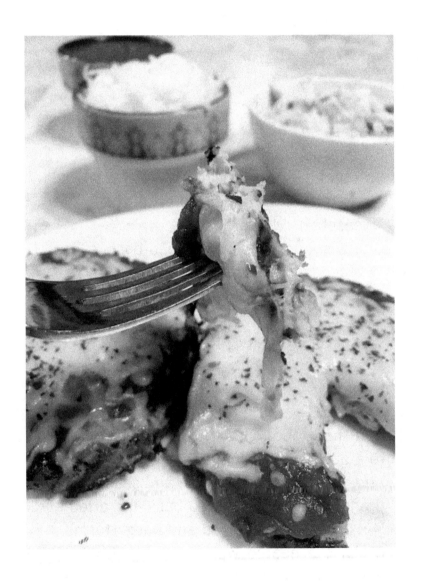

Italian Chicken and Basil Chaffles

Preparation time: 10 minutes
Cooking Time: 7–9 Minutes
Servings: 2

Ingredients:
- Batter
- ½ pound ground chicken
- 4 eggs
- 3 tablespoons tomato sauce
- Salt and pepper to taste
- 1 cup grated mozzarella cheese
- 1 teaspoon dried oregano
- 3 tablespoons freshly chopped basil leaves
- ½ teaspoon dried garlic
- Other
- 2 tablespoons butter to brush the waffle maker
- ¼ cup tomato sauce for serving
- 1 tablespoon freshly chopped basil for serving

Directions:
1. Preheat the waffle maker.
2. Add the ground chicken, eggs and tomato sauce to a bowl and season with salt and pepper.
3. Add the mozzarella cheese and season with dried oregano, freshly chopped basil and dried garlic.
4. Mix until fully combined and batter forms.
5. Brush the heated waffle maker with butter and add a few tablespoons of the chaffle batter.
6. Close the lid and cook for about 7–9 minutes depending on your waffle maker.

7. Repeat with the rest of the batter.
8. Serve with tomato sauce and freshly chopped basil on top.

Nutrition: Calories: 253, Fat: 17 g, Protein: 11 g, Carbohydrates: 21 g, Fiber – 2 g

Beef Meatballs on Chaffle

Preparation time: 10 minutes
Cooking Time:20 Minutes
Servings: 2
Ingredients:
- Batter
- 4 eggs
- 2½ cups grated gouda cheese
- ¼ cup heavy cream
- Salt and pepper to taste
- 1 spring onion, finely chopped
- Beef meatballs
- 1 pound ground beef
- Salt and pepper to taste
- 2 teaspoons Dijon mustard
- 1 spring onion, finely chopped
- 5 tablespoons almond flour
- 2 tablespoons butter
- Other
- 2 tablespoons cooking spray to brush the waffle maker
- 2 tablespoons freshly chopped parsley

Directions:
1. Preheat the waffle maker.
2. Add the eggs, grated gouda cheese, heavy cream, salt and pepper and finely chopped spring onion to a bowl.
3. Mix until combined and batter forms.

4. Brush the heated waffle maker with cooking spray and add a few tablespoons of the batter.
5. Close the lid and cook for about 7 minutes depending on your waffle maker.
6. Meanwhile, mix the ground beef meat, salt and pepper, Dijon mustard, chopped spring onion and almond flour in a large bowl.
7. Form small meatballs with your hands.
8. Heat the butter in a nonstick frying pan and cook the beef meatballs for about 3–4 minutes on each side.
9. Serve each chaffle with a couple of meatballs and some freshly chopped parsley on top.

Nutrition: Calories: 159, Fat: 7 g, Protein: 9 g, Carbohydrates: 15 g, Fiber: 0.8 g

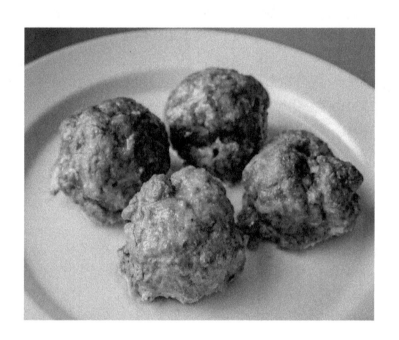

CPSIA information can be obtained
at www.ICGtesting.com
Printed in the USA
BVHW092049190421
605311BV00002B/163